An Adventure A Day

a program to

promote one's

physical and mental core

by

C. D. Gryphon

This is dedicated to my

family and friends who supported

me along with all of my adventures over the years

Table of Contents

Very important

The words in the following pages may inspire you to alter or make changes to your lifestyle. Therefore it is very important to consult your physician prior to making any changes to your lifestyle to minimize the risk of adverse affects.

History

* One can learn a lot from their elders *

I spent most of my summers as a kid visiting both sets of my grandparents. We would go for walks, work on jigsaw puzzles and do word puzzles on a daily basis. Both sets of my grandparents lived good and long lives.

***

The *An Adventure A Day* idea started a few summers ago when I was between jobs. I had a free summer to do stuff and I was hanging out with my best friend (who was a teacher and had summers off too). We would do daily activities such as hike and bike whenever we could. One day, while getting ready for a hike, my friend's wife asked "Why are you going out hiking again when you just did a hike yesterday?" My answer was "Today is a different day. And we need to have an adventure a day." That's how the daily adventures started.

After many years and many adventures, with lots of work, using a lifetime's worth of knowledge and experiences, and with a crazy desire to further develop *An Adventure A Day*, the project was finally completed. It's an idea that I believe in and that is simple yet effective to help promote a strong and healthy body. It has taken me many years to get to this final version of which I am very happy to share. I just hope that some people will benefit from *An Adventure A Day* as I have, and as I still do.

Background

Imagine that a person is made up of three main components. Just like the three sides of a triangle- 'a triangle of life' so to speak. These three components, or sides, are the body, the mind and the spirit. It is best when each component, or side is optimized, or maximized, therefore ensuring a good strong triangle just as one would have a good strong body (the body here refers to the entire individual).

The body is the physical core, or physical component of a person. The body is made up of muscles, tissues, bones and organs. It is best when the body is exercised and is active on a regular basis.

The mind is the mental core, or mental component of an individual. Imagine the mind as the mental muscle of an individual. The mind needs be exercised just like any other muscle in order to be in its optimum condition. The best mental exercises are activities that inspire and challenge an individual.

The spirit is what motivates or drives an individual. The spirit component can be seen as a broad personal aspect of which may be comprised of a single or a multitude of factors that might include religious beliefs (or not), ideals, family, and/or goals, but for *An Adventure A Day*, the spirit is the personal drive or motivation of an individual. It is important to have a strong spirit. It is the third side in 'the triangle of life' and is just as important as the two other sides- the body and the mind.

Ideally, each of the three components (the body, the mind and the spirit) can be optimized without negatively affecting the others.

What is *An Adventure A Day*?

An Adventure A Day is simply that. For one to have an adventure a day.

* The purpose of *An Adventure A Day* is to promote the physical and mental core of an individual through activities called Adventures on a daily basis *

These adventures will fit into one of two categories- physical and mental.

Physical adventures are meant to promote the physical component of a person. Physical adventures always involve some sort of physical activity in one form or another.

Mental adventures are meant to promote the mental component of a person. Mental adventures are meant to inspire, challenge, and overall use the mind. Most mental adventures involve games, puzzles, social interactions, physical activities with mental components, and in some cases may involve relaxation.

An Adventure A Day is intended to apply to the body and the mind but not the spirit (however the spirit can benefit from one's adventures). Anyone can do *An Adventure A Day*, regardless of the basis of their spirit. Because the spirit varies from person to person, each person will promote their spirit their own way. One's spiritual component may influence which adventures one does, but it should not prevent one from doing any physical or mental adventures at all. Therefore, the basis of one's spiritual component should not prevent one from doing *An Adventure A Day*.

An Adventure A Day is also meant to separate oneself from the daily routines of one's life. These daily routines are not bad by any means, however one's daily routines can inhibit inspiration and creative thought, prevent one from relaxing, can cause stress, or in the worst of situations could lead to physical or mental ailments. One's daily routines can also distract oneself, therefore reducing the benefits of one's adventures.   It is best when a person is focused on his or her adventure and when all distractions are minimized.

One needs both a strong physical and mental core to succeed, especially if one is determined to live a long and productive life. And if a long and productive life may not be a goal, *An Adventure A Day* could help one's current situation by promoting one's physical and mental core.

In the following pages, the *An Adventure A Day* program to help promote one's physical and mental core will be explained in more detail.

Getting the most out of *An Adventure A Day*

In addition to having physical and mental adventures, one can benefit further by fulfilling two other components that are considered to be important in the *An Adventure A Day* program. The two other components are the Variety and Bonus components.

A person that seeks to fulfill both the Variety and Bonus components could end up with stronger physical and mental sides of the 'triangle of life' than a person that did not.

The Variety component

What good would it be to have a body that is physically fit when you do not have the mental wits to match? Or if you were mentally sharp but lacked the physical abilities to let you get out and about. This is especially important as one gets older. Both the physical and the mental components of an individual are needed for one to have a good strong body, and this is best fulfilled by doing both physical and mental adventures.

In *An Adventure A Day*, the variety component is comprised of two subcomponents-subcomponent #1-one needs both physical and mental adventures (as noted above), and subcomponent #2- there has to be variety within one's physical and mental adventures (noted below).

If one just did the same activity over and over then one would not really be getting a well balanced program. One *An Adventure A Day* theory is if one did a variety of activities, that person would benefit more than a person that did the same activity over and over. Physically, one should benefit more from a program with a variety of physical adventures as more muscle groups are exercised rather than repeating a single type of physical activity that exercises a few select muscle groups. A good physical variety program exercises more of the body's muscles so a larger portion of the body benefits more. A physical program with variety can then be viewed as a great way to optimize the physical component of the body. The same can be said about mental adventures. The ideal outcome of doing mental adventures is increased mental activity, and this can be best fulfilled with a variety of mental activities. If one just does the same mental activity all the time, then one is not really challenging oneself, the creativity and the inspiration components are not gained, and one does not benefit as much as a person who has a good variety of mental activities. Variety within one's physical and mental programs is important as variety helps maximize the benefits from one's adventures.

So in *An Adventure A Day*, doing adventures are good, but for one to benefit the most from the *An Adventure A Day* program, one should do both physical and mental adventures in addition to having variety within one's physical and mental adventure programs.

The Bonus component

There will always be special events, circumstances, or milestones of which an individual can benefit more than that of a normal adventure. These special events, circumstances, or milestones in *An Adventure A Day* are called bonuses. Bonuses can be adventures or bonuses might involve adventures. Bonuses can be either physically or mentally based. A bonus can be a physical challenge such as participating in a race, or it can be a mental inspirational event such as going to a museum or a zoo. Overall it is meant to inspire and/or challenge an individual more than just a regular adventure.

Since bonuses can be adventures, if the bonus meets the requirements of an adventure then one can count the bonus both as an adventure and as a bonus.

The details behind the *An Adventure a Day* program

A good boss of mine used to promote the practice of 'keep it simple'. The 'keep it simple' ideology can lead one to think 'the simpler things are, then the more likely a person will stick with it'. So simplicity can be a key for success and long term program participation.

An Adventure A Day is a program with a simple design that is based on adventures. Just do and record your adventures. The overall program and the tracking of those adventures also uses the 'keep it simple' ideology.

When it comes to *An Adventure A Day*, tracking one's progress is as easy as ABC, or in this case AVB.

A - Adventures

V - Variety

B - Bonuses

In *An Adventure A Day*, one will simply count the adventures and the bonuses, and see if the variety component is met on a weekly basis.

It is recommended that one gets a calendar or a calendar program to record one's progress. It's ok to not record one's progress if one just wants to have daily adventures. However, one could benefit more from *An Adventure A Day* if one simply records one's adventures and progress.

Important note regarding recording one's progress- one just needs enough space to note all of the adventures and a place to add up the results on a weekly basis. This means that any small calendar would do. And the more notes one records, the better the chances are that one will benefit more from one's *An Adventure A Day* program.

So what notes is one supposed to record? Please read further.

What counts as an Adventure?

All adventures will be of two categories- physical or mental.

Each adventure will count as one (1) Adventure point.

Below is a simple list of adventures.

Physical adventures

Physical adventures are meant to promote the physical component of a person. Physical adventures always involve some sort of physical activity in one form or another.

All physical adventures should last a minimum of 1 hour. If a person runs for 5 hours it still is considered one (1) physical Adventure point.

Examples are:

Walking

Running

Hiking

Biking (road, mountain, etc)

Skiing (x-country, downhill, etc)

Snowboarding

Snowshoeing

Paddleboarding

Windsurfing

Kayaking

Canoeing

Swimming / Snorkeling / Diving

Rock climbing / Bouldering

Martial Arts

Tennis

Racquetball

Squash

Table tennis/ping pong

Backpacking

Team sports (football, baseball, softball, basketball, hockey, etc.)

Gym workouts

Mental adventures

Mental adventures are meant to promote the mental component of a person. Mental adventures are meant to inspire, challenge, and overall use the mind. Most mental adventures involve games, puzzles, social interactions, physical activities with mental components, and in some cases may involve relaxation.

Mental adventures should last a minimum of 1 hour.

Examples are:

Jigsaw puzzling

Games (chess, checkers, poker, Scrabble, Monopoly, card games, board games, etc.) (No video games.) The games are meant to be played with other people. The games should involve some sort of thought or strategy. Includes family game night.

Visit an aquarium, zoo, museum or art gallery

See a show, opera, symphony, live music, concert or play

Take a tour (a tourist attraction tour, a city tour, etc.)

Finish reading a book or a novel

Play a musical instrument (try to play with another person, a group, or a band)

Karaoke

See a movie in a theater (only count once per week)

Do a social event with friends or family (away from home) (Brunch, lunch, dinner, guys night out, girls night out, etc.) (only count once per week)

Learn and make a new meal (only count once per week)

Start a new hobby (can be physical or mental hobby) (the first 3 sessions can be counted as mental adventures due to learning a new skill)

Visit a festival or a farmers market (art and wine festivals, Octoberfest, etc) (only count once per week)

Meditation

Receive a professional massage (1 hour minimum) or spa day for relaxation (only count once per week)

Attend one of your kid's events (sports event, play, etc.)

Physical or Mental adventures

The following adventures can be counted as either physical or mental adventures since they can promote either the physical or the mental component of an individual.

Again, each adventure should last a minimum of 1 hour.

Dancing

Tai Chi

Yoga

Golf (Be your own caddie if possible)

Minigolf (only count once per week)

Archery

Fencing

Billiards/pool games

Volunteer (mental or physical activity)

Visit a theme park or carnival (with rides, roller coasters, water slides, etc) (Disneyland, Six flags, water theme parks, etc.)

Flying a kite

Sailing

Horseback riding

Hunting

Fishing

Create your own adventure

There are a lot of adventures that are not listed in the above in physical or mental categories. Feel free to incorporate your own adventures into either the physical or mental categories as long as the adventure fits into the physical or mental category definition.

Enjoy your adventure

If you go to the zoo, do you leave after an hour? Even though an adventure is supposed to last a minimum of one hour, it is highly recommended to extend that adventure as long as you can. Don't just stop at one hour to get that Adventure point. You are already doing the adventure, so just do it as long as possible. This is not a contest of who finishes first, rather you are the only winner and you get out of it what you put into it. So enjoy your adventure and try not to rush it if you don't have to.

Mini adventures

There are times when a little activity can go a long way. Some activities or adventures, when performed frequently (on a daily basis if possible), their act, even though for a short time, can be more beneficial than doing the same activity or adventure, once for an hour. These short activities, or adventures, are called mini adventures.

Mini adventures are a great way to incorporate a short activity or adventure into a busy schedule.

Mini adventures are considered to be important to the *An Adventure A Day* program and are highly recommended as the results can be more beneficial than just a single adventure!

Here are three types of mini adventures:

Stretch for 15 minutes a day for a minimum of 5 days (perform everyday if possible). This will count as one (1) physical Adventure point. Can be counted once per week.

Puzzle for 15 minutes per day for a minimum of 5 days (perform everyday if possible). This includes daily puzzles, crosswords, searchwords, Sudoku, etc. This will count as one (1) mental Adventure point. Can be counted once per week.

Walk 4 times for a minimum of 30 minutes each time. This can be done multiple times per day or over many days, but can only be counted within a week's time. Each 4-30 minute session counts as one (1) physical Adventure point. This can be repeated many times. If one walks 8-30 minute walks over a week's time then that person can claim two (2) physical Adventure points. This is ideal for those who have limited time throughout the day and only have few opportunities for adventures. It's also great for dog walkers! Additionally, frequent small walks throughout the day can boost one's circulation, especially when one is not physically active for prolonged periods of time.

Create your own mini adventure

Do the same adventure for a minimum of 30 minutes 4 times a week and count it as one (1) Adventure point. This is just like the above walk 30 minutes mini adventure but applies to any adventure. This is best for people who don't have the hour to spend yet want to still do some sort of adventure or activity. Short daily gym workouts easily meet this category. The create your own mini adventures can be physical or mental.

Multi-adventure day

A person can always do more than one adventure a day. There is no limit to how many adventures one can do in a day. Feel free and try and do as many adventures as you can. It is encouraged to do as many adventures as possible.

Variety points

Variety points are earned on a weekly basis and one can earn a maximum of one (1) Variety point per week. This means a maximum of 52 Variety points per year can be earned.

As stated earlier, there are two subcomponents that need to be met for one to earn the weekly Variety point.

Variety subcomponent #1- one needs both physical and mental adventures. One needs to complete 7 adventures in a week of which 4 Adventure points need to be from physical adventures and 3 Adventure points need to be from mental adventures. An optional challenge- one who works a physical job, or who is very athletic, then the rule can be reversed and 3 Adventure points need to be from physical adventures and 4 Adventure points need to be from mental adventures to earn the weekly Variety point.

Variety subcomponent #2- there has to be variety within one's physical and mental adventures. One can't count more than 2 of the same type of Adventure points towards the Variety point. So to count 3 Adventure points one has to do 3 adventures in 2 different types of activities. Or one can do 3 different types of adventures once each. For example, one can run 3 times in a week but one can only count 2 physical Adventure points of running towards the Variety point (one can still count 3 Adventure points for the runs). So if one needs to count 4 Adventure points towards the Variety point, then one has to do 2 different types of adventures, each done twice. Or 3 different types of adventures, with one type of adventure done twice. Or 4 different types of adventures, each done once. Bottom line- one can't count the same adventure more than twice towards the Variety point.

Mini adventures can be counted towards the variety subcomponents.

Bonuses

Bonuses are special events, circumstances, or milestones that inspire and/or challenge an individual more than just a regular adventure. The following bonuses can only be counted for one (1) Bonus point each per year unless noted otherwise. Not all bonuses are adventures. However, if the bonus is an adventure, then one can count it both as an adventure and a bonus.

The Grand Slam- do a different adventure per day for a week for a total of 7 different adventures (do not count any mini adventures). Make sure the variety component is met (4 physical/3 mental or 3 physical/4 mental). Then also do the puzzle, stretch and walk mini adventures. Outcome is 10 Adventure points and 1 Variety point. (The Grand Slam can be counted once per week)

1 Bonus point for every domestic state visited for pleasure

1 Bonus point for every international country visited for pleasure

Visit and tour your state's capital

Visit and tour your nation's capital

1 Bonus point for every other state capital that you visit and tour

1 Bonus point for every race (5k walk, etc.) that you participate in

1 Bonus point for every National Park or National Monument visited

1 Bonus point for every State Park visited

Visit the largest body of water such as the ocean, lake, river, etc. within 200 miles

Visit the top of the highest peak within 200 miles

Visit an aquarium or a zoo

Visit an art gallery or a museum

See a show, opera, play, symphony, live music (that is not part of a kid's performance)

Volunteer 1 day - volunteering is a great way to get involved with one's community

Support one of your kid's events (game, play, etc)

Take a special vacation with just your spouse (anniversary, special occasion, etc. without any kids)

Take a vacation without your spouse (overnighter, etc)

Do a good deed for a stranger

Learn and make 6 new meals

Read 6 novels

De-tech for 24 hours (Do not use any electronic equipment for a day (phones for emergency, lights, clocks, emergency items ok.) Use pedal power or walk. Must be voluntary, not a sick day, etc.)

Create your own bonus

Just like 'Create your own adventure', if there is a special event, a circumstance, or a milestone that inspired and/or challenged you more than just a regular adventure, then go ahead and count it as a bonus for a Bonus point- but count it only once. You can create new bonuses but you can only use each once. And make sure your bonus is extraordinary. For example, a backpacking trip is a good adventure, but a 50 mile backpacking trip (which is like a marathon of backpacking) is a bonus. Visiting a World Heritage site would also be a good event to merit a Bonus point.

Recording your progress

So what does one record?

Just record the adventure after it happens!

It is highly recommended to record one's adventures that one does on a daily basis. Then at the end of the week, one should add up the adventures and the mini adventures, note whether the variety component was met, and finally, add up all the bonuses. Then one should add the Adventure, Variety and Bonus points to the year-to-date totals. So, on the last day of the week, one should know the number of Adventure, Variety and Bonus points for the week and year-to-date.

Helpful recording hints

In my calendar, I note a 'P' if I did puzzles that day. I also use 'S' for stretches and 'W' for walks. Then I write down what adventure(s) I did that day. And I circle or mark the adventure or event if it is a bonus. I try to do this on a daily basis. At the end of the week (Sunday is the last day of the week in my calendar), I add up the adventures and the mini adventures, I see if I met the variety component, and finally I add up the bonuses. Then I add them to last week's totals to get the year-to-date values.

Scoring/rating yourself

If one does an adventure a day then one would have 365 Adventure (physical and mental) points in a year (366 for leap years). There really is no limit to the amount of Adventure points one can earn, especially if one does more than one adventure a day and mini adventures too.

The variety component has a maximum of 52 Variety points. One point per week.

The bonus component has no maximum. However, just like adventures, the more the better.

As for what score is ideal for *An Adventure A Day* - there really is no ideal score. There is no great, average, or bad. There is no rating system at all! The points are more of a tracking system than a rating system. The higher the score the better. You are not competing against other individuals, rather you are the sole person that benefits from your actions. You get out of it what you put into it. Try and record your Adventure, Variety and Bonus scores over time. Plus, with enough data and some statistical formulas/tools, one might identify trends with one's adventures over time (such as types and frequency of adventures). See what you can come up with.

Just doing an adventure a day does not guarantee any Variety or Bonus points. Variety points are earned from having a well balanced program. Bonus points are earned from doing special events, circumstances, or milestones. As stated earlier, a person that seeks to fulfill both the Variety and Bonus components could have stronger physical and mental sides of the 'triangle of life' than one that did not.

Even though there is no rating system, a score of 469 Adventures points (470 for a leap year) and 52 Variety points over a year would be warrant for a congratulations and a pat on the back. (the 469/470 comes from an adventure a day plus the stretch and puzzle mini adventures per week). If you need a goal, then use these numbers.

FAQ - Are there any exceptions due to illness, injury, travel, family, etc? The simple answer to this is NO! Try and do whatever you can. If you are sick, then relax and get better. Maybe read a book or do other non-stressful mental or physical adventures. If you have an injury, do whatever physical or mental adventures you can, concentrate on your rehabilitation/physical therapy exercises, maybe do more low impact physical adventures, but just do whatever you can.

Overall it might seem that there are a lot of rules, but when you look at the An *Adventure A Day* program and try it out, then it should seem to be a simple program. Just like checkers- there are some rules, but once you start playing it, it is one of the easiest games around. In my opinion, *An Adventure A Day* is a simple and easy program, as easy as checkers. Plus you are always the winner!

Progress checks

Progress checks are a good way to optimize an ongoing program by using feedback from past and current events to possibly alter future events. Progress checks do not need to be complicated, rather progress checks can be simple exercises or reviews. One type of a progress check is a self evaluation (or self review). And a good time for a self evaluation progress check is at the end of the week when one is adding up one's weekly adventure totals. A few things to note at that time would be:

- Weekly recap of activities
- Did you do what you wanted to do?
- Next week's suggestions/goals

Overall this is meant to be a simple exercise of which it should take a few seconds to a few minutes to complete. The progress check can be done mentally, and one can note the results in their calendar if one wishes.

One can always add more criteria to review during the progress checks.

Progress checks can be done as often as one wishes. Other good times for progress checks are at the end of the year when one adds up all of the year-to-date totals of Adventures, Variety and Bonus points, or at other milestone dates.

Goals

Even though *An Adventure A Day*'s main purpose is to have an adventure a day, it is recommended to have a goal to help one focus those adventures (an example is to participate in a race so one must then train for it), or to have a goal to look forward to something (such as a trip/vacation). An additional reason for having a goal is to introduce a positive reward system which one will have to work on, to reach, or achieve the goal. The success from the accomplishment of reaching, or achieving the goal can also help build up one's confidence. The goal can be a minor or a major goal. The goal should be achievable within the year. After the goal is accomplished, celebrate, then move on to the next goal.

How much will *An Adventure A Day* cost me?

With the exception of the cost of this book, *An Adventure A Day* should be totally cost free! There's no special equipment, membership fees, dues or hidden costs. One can use any free calendar or notebook and a pen or pencil to record and add up one's adventures. Adventures shouldn't have any extra costs when associated with *An Adventure A Day*. The only costs are costs directly associated with one's adventures (there are always costs associated with activities such as hiking boots, a bike or other gear). So you only pay into *An Adventure A Day* what you want and you benefit 100% from your investment. You do not need to purchase anything extra to do A*n Adventure A Day.*

When to start *An Adventure A Day*

Now is a great time to start. Don't even finish the book! Just go out there and do an adventure! Then record your adventure and then finish reading *An Adventure A Day*.

A person can start *An Adventure A Day* just about anytime throughout their life. (Please check with a physician prior to making any changes to your lifestyle to minimize the risk of adverse affects.) Ideally, *An Adventure A Day* can be followed throughout one's life so it can be seen as a 'life' routine. *An Adventure A Day* should be able to be performed with other training or diet regimens too (please confirm with a physician). Therefore, *An Adventure A Day* should be able to be started anytime in one's life regardless of what a person is doing at that stage of their life.

****

Recommended principles for *An Adventure A Day*

An Adventure A Day is a pretty simple program. If one just followed *An Adventure A Day*, then ideally one should have a good physical and mental core. However, there are some principles that *An Adventure A Day* recommends, and they are listed below.

Diet

One's diet is very important and should not be taken for granted. A good diet can help boost one's metabolism and energy levels, it can affect emotions, and most important, it can influence both the mental and physical well-being of a person. There are a plethora of different diets out there with each diet targeting a specific person, food group or cause. Additionally, people have different dietary requirements which can be based on a multitude of factors, including genetics, allergies, current health issues, age, and gender. Also, one should factor in the current metabolic requirements of one's body in addition to the energy requirements for adventures and/or activities (upcoming events- carbo-loading, current events- maintaining energy levels, or completed events- recovery). So given all of the variables, it is really impossible to promote any one type of diet.

* An Adventure a Day does not promote any one specific type of diet *

Even though *An Adventure a Day* does not promote any particular diet, *An Adventure a Day* does have a few recommendations regarding one's diet:

- Check with your doctor for nutritional recommendations based upon your current physical condition.

- Eat a balanced diet.
- Eat fruits and vegetables (two easily overlooked food groups).
- Make sure your body has all of its building blocks. Take vitamins and supplements as needed and recommended.
- Eat fresh foods over processed foods.
- Eat foods rich in special components over dietary supplements. When looking for a special component in your diet, and if you have a choice between a food or a supplement, go with the food. The processing to create a dietary supplement might not create a fully equal product.
- Listen to your stomach (body). If you are craving a food, this could be your body telling you that you need to fulfill a dietary requirement. So cravings can help satisfy nutritional or caloric deficiencies of which one is not aware of.

The term 'diet' does not just refer to what types of food to eat. It can also refer to the portions or amounts taken in. The portions of a diet can be just as important as the content itself. As stated above, eat a balanced diet. This does not mean to eat equal portions of each group, rather it means eat appropriate portions of each group per what your body needs. Portions can be easily overlooked, especially in today's times when restaurants offer generous meals to its patrons. So eat according to what your body needs and not always what's on your plate.

One's diet is one of the easiest changes one can make to their lifestyle of which the benefits can be quickly and easily noticed.

One's diet is very important and should not be neglected!

Hydration

Hydration is a very important factor to one's well-being and one's hydration levels can quickly affect one's physical and mental components. A lot of people are not sufficiently hydrated throughout a normal day. Most people only think about hydration during an adventure or an activity. This is the wrong way to address hydration. Hydration must be addressed throughout the entire day regardless if one is active or not. When a person is not properly hydrated, then he or she is not performing at optimum levels. So if you are not properly hydrated, a few extra ounces of water throughout the day could be all that is needed to bring you to optimum levels.

So drink enough fluids to be properly hydrated. Substitute water for sodas and other sugary drinks. If tired of water, drink hot tea, iced tea or even plain coffee (please choose your teas and coffees wisely as they may have unwanted ingredients).

Hydration is very important!

Sleep

Wouldn't it be wonderful to wake up every morning on your own after a good night's rest and you are fully energized for the upcoming day? Sadly, not everyone has this luxury. Most people use an alarm to wake up, and then they start their day whether they are fully rested or not. People often think that they can get by with less sleep than what the body needs so sleep is often neglected or overlooked.   People often think that they can make up sleep at a later time too. Some people force themselves to stay awake via stimulants (caffeine, etc.) or even by increasing one's energy intake (sugar, food, etc.). Sleep is an essential body function and is very important to the well-being of a person. The lack of sleep affects both the physical and mental components of a person. Lack of sleep can cause chemical imbalances in the body. Lack of sleep can affect appetites, and possibly even cause weight gain for those that choose to consume food to provide energy to stay alert past normal times. Sleep is also the time that the body uses to regenerate and heal itself. Sleep is very important! So don't take sleep for granted and get enough sleep per your body's needs (each person has different sleep requirements).

Sleep not just applies to the interval between night and morning. Sometimes the body just needs a little break, a rest or a pause during the day. These little breaks, rests or pauses can turn into naps. Some people refer to these naps as 'catnaps' or 'powernaps'. It's amazing that a 20 minute nap can energize a person more than a stimulant. Short naps at the right times (usually when the body is exhausted, fatigued, etc) can be a great way to help reenergize the body.

Sleep is an essential body function and one's sleep habits are very important and should not be neglected!

Take that extra step

Why not take every possible chance to increase your fitness. It's easy, just keep moving and avoid certain things.

* Technology can be great but it can also rob people of valuable exercise *

One great way to boost one's fitness is to avoid using escalators, moving walkways (often located in airports) and elevators, and to walk and take the stairs whenever possible. This can easily be done in places such as airports (airport travel days usually involve lots of inactivity as one tends to sit for prolonged periods of time on planes and in the airport itself), malls and multi-story buildings.

When parking for an event, why waste time looking for the nearest spot and just park a little further away (make sure to park in a safe location) and walk the extra distance to your destination. Not only does this action increase your fitness, but it might also decrease some stress by eliminating the game of looking and fighting for that perfect close parking spot. An extra bonus is that it may decrease the chances of your car getting damaged by strangers and other vehicles.

Bottom line- it all comes down to picking the path with a few extra steps for the sole purpose of increasing your fitness.

So take that extra step when you can!

Flexibility and balance

Flexibility and balance are often overlooked and taken for granted.

The more you move, the better. Try and stay flexible because one's flexibility can decrease as one gets older. This is why the daily stretches, if performed, are so valuable. This is why doing physical adventures are essential to longevity. This is where every little bit of physical activity adds up. And the more physical adventures one does, especially with proper warm-ups and warm-downs, the better.

Good balance can improve one's physical motions. Think about a ballerina. A ballerina with bad balance would likely use more energy trying to maintain good form and would be more likely to make a mistake. A ballerina with good balance would have more graceful moves and would also use less energy when executing those moves.   Even though not everyone aspires to be a ballerina, balance is important to everyone. Balance is essential to many physical activities such as bicycling, rock climbing and dancing. Good balance could help prevent or reduce injuries. If one falls, trips or stumbles, a person with good balance might have a better chance of recovering from the event and end up not falling, tripping or stumbling. If injury did occur, there is a possibility that the injury was reduced due to good balance.

There are a lot of adventures (dance, tai chi, yoga and rock climbing) that promote flexibility and balance. So be aware of which adventures promote flexibility and balance and try and remember that when not doing those adventures to possibly try and add a flexibility and balance promoting adventure or activity into your overall routine.

Be spontaneous and try new things

Being spontaneous, trying new activities or visiting new places are good for multiple reasons.

Mentally (with physical or mental adventures), it can make one 'think outside of the box' and it can give one a challenge with a different activity or scenario. Or it may inspire just by introducing something new.

Physically, it may involve a new physical adventure, therefore exercising different muscles. Or with regular physical adventures with a new location or route, one would then have to be more alert, physically and mentally, due to possible unknown obstacles that may be around the corner.

Overall, it is good to try something new or different every once in a while.

Involve the family

Family is very important and should never be neglected. One can always have family members join in when attempting an adventure.

An Adventure A Day is also a wonderful way to spend time with kids. Why does one need to go to a formal performance such as a play or the ballet, when one can see a performance of a child? Also, some adventures can be done with a child. Incorporate your children in your activity. Toss your kid in a stroller and go for a walk, a run or a ride. Play a game of mini golf with your children, take them to the beach/water, and just enjoy the day. Go to a zoo or a museum. Kids will benefit from the experience as you do too. Learn and play games with kids. Not only will you benefit by doing an adventure, but your child can benefit too.

You benefit from every action that you do

Do you just do adventures and nothing else?

Do you just benefit from your adventures and from nothing else?

Adventures are great, however one's physical and mental core benefits from all actions one does. Every little bit counts. Doing a mini adventure, walking that extra 100 feet or just taking the stairs, you benefit from all of your actions. So one does not just benefit from one's adventures, rather one benefits from everything one does. Whether one counts it or not.

* every little bit matters *

That is why just doing adventures are good, but adding extra actions are great. Get the most of your actions!

Be safe and be prepared

Why bother to get the most out of your life if you are not safe with your adventures and you never make it to the next adventure, or to the next day, the next year, or a nice old age? Be safe and be prepared for your adventures. A few minutes preparing for your adventure (or an emergency) can save time and resources when the unexpected happens.

Every adventure has different safety and preparatory requirements. Preparing for an adventure can include a multitude of factors to include checking out the details of the adventure (weather, map, terrain, location) or important times to note (when does the show start or when are you to meet others) to carrying the proper gear. Being informed and/or prepared can possibly save you time and may reduce stress if something unexpected happens.

As stated above, proper preparation also includes having the proper gear. If you expect rain- bring a rain jacket or an umbrella, lots of sun- bring sun tan lotion, lots of bugs- bring a bug net or use bug repellant. Overall, a small bit of preparation can make the adventure more bearable during stressful situations.

An Adventure A Day recommends to always carry a whistle, regardless of the adventure or the location. A whistle is a small, easy to operate, low tech device that could help a person out when a bad situation arises. A whistle is a great device to call for help. A whistle can be heard when used in crowded areas. A whistle can signal where you are and a whistle can be heard over long distances, and therefore is great when one needs to signal others far away, such as when one is in the outdoors (or the open ocean such as for divers). And regardless of what part of the world you are in, or what language is spoken, a whistle is mostly regarded as a signal/alert device.

One should always be safe with one's adventures. Do not take unnecessary risks and use good judgment in adventures and unexpected events.

****

The 5% theory

At a minimum, if one does an adventure a day, in essence that person is dedicating 5% or less of their total existence to adventures. 5% is not a large amount, rather it is a very small amount of the whole. So just doing *An Adventure A Day* could prove more beneficial than any other activity for the same amount of time (except sleep).

Do whatever you can

Not everyone has time to have an adventure a day. So do whatever you can and incorporate as many recommended principles and ideas you can into your routine. Record your adventures if you choose to. You benefit from every action that you do whether it is an adventure or not and whether you record it or not. Plus you may not feel all the effort that you put into your routine, but you probably will appreciate it over your lifetime as you get older. So go out there and have an adventure and do whatever you can!

****

About the author C.D. Gryphon

I was born and raised in the San Francisco Bay Area of California. I didn't always stay in the SF Bay Area but I was always drawn back to it, for it has great terrain for outdoor activities and it has great opportunities for work. I had a good childhood. I've always tried to be active both physically and mentally. I studied biology, chemistry and oceanography in college. And I worked in the sciences for many years. Overall, I'm just a normal person.

My accomplishments and my track record - at a minimum, I try to do an adventure a day (I have a pretty good success rate and good AVB scores). Most of my adventures involve walking, hiking, skiing (when there's snow), biking, puzzling and exploring new places.

****

The end

Adventures over time

Year	Adventures	Variety	Bonuses
2013			
2014			
2015			
2016			
2017			
2018			
2019			
2020			
2021			
2022			
2023			
2024			
2025